RELAXING IN THE HIGH DESERT

A meditative story to massage your body
and relax your mind

BOOKS IN THE NATUREBODY® SERIES

—

Walking in an Ancient Forest

Camping Under the Night Sky

Relaxing by a Waterfall

A Peaceful Winter Ski

Swimming in a Tropical Sea

A Healing Coastal Walk

Relaxing in the High Desert

A Spirited Mountain Hike

The complete
NatureBody® Connection
program is available at

www.aquaterramassage.com

Relaxing in the
HIGH
DESERT

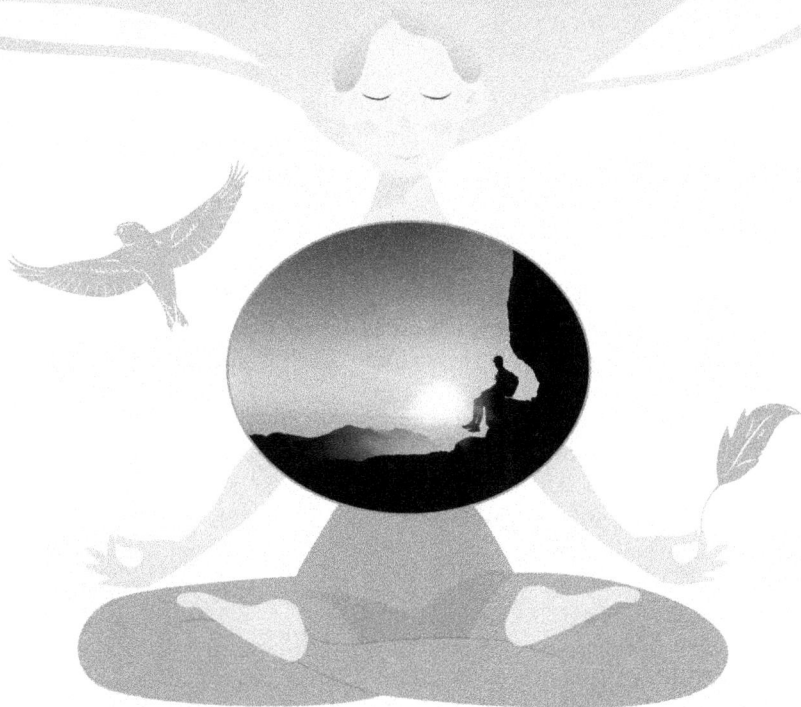

A meditative story to massage your body
and relax your mind

ERIK KRIPPNER *and* FAYE KRIPPNER

ISBN: 978-1-959772-02-6

Cover art provided by Envato Elements. Cover design by Faye Krippner and Erik Krippner.

Release Date for First Printed Edition 2023.

Media Inquiries: If you would like to contact the authors, please send an email to press@aquaterramassage.com.

Faye Krippner, B.A., LMT and Erik Krippner, B.S., LMT have been licensed by the Oregon Board of Massage Therapy since 2003. Oregon License Numbers: 10233 & 10234

Experience the entire NatureBody® Connection at
www.aquaterramassage.com

For the wisdom seekers.

May you
hear songs in the wind
and
see stories in the clouds.

Index of Reflections

Arching to Release Our Shoulders 6

The Core of Movement 8

On Grounding 10

The Grace of an Antelope 14

Pivoting From Your Hips 16

Finding Your Balance. 18

The Strength of a Tree 22

On Aging 24

Nurturing Yourself 26

On Breathing Freely 30

The Breathing Planet 32

The Ideal Bedroll 36

Effortless Breathing 38

On Eternity 40

Contents

HOW TO USE THIS BOOK   IX

INTRODUCTION   1

BETWEEN EARTH AND SKY   5
Stretching and Grounding

SPIRIT OF THE ANTELOPE   13
Agility and Freedom of the Hips

WISDOM OF THE LAND   21
Aging with Grace

WIND SONG AND CLOUD STORIES   29
Breathing Meditation

TRANSITION TO EVENING   35
Full Body Meditation

GRATITUDE   43
A Blessing From the High Desert

ACKNOWLEDGMENTS   45

NOTES   47

JOURNAL   51

ABOUT THE AUTHORS   94

How to Use This Book

Humans have lived in balance with our bodies and the earth for 2.6 million years. Our bodies are designed for this planet. It is natural to walk on uneven ground, climb mountains, run long distances, swim, and most of all, to deeply breathe fresh air. Our wild planet heals and strengthens us by making us more flexible and fluid.

Your body is born of this earth. Earth is here to support you. Unfortunately, the stresses of life pull us off balance, and can leave us feeling physically sore and mentally anxious. This creative journey into relaxation is a way to remember your natural balance and create new muscle memories.

As massage therapists, we understand how a relaxed body feels: how it breathes, how it moves, how it is balanced in space. This NatureBody® massage story shares the full spectrum of massage: body, mind and spirit. Our intention is to empower you to find healing within yourself.

Visualization can have powerful effects on your body.[1] In this guided visualization, you will exercise your mind and imagination to deeply relax and bring your body back to center.

If you are injured or your ability to move is limited, then visualization is even more important! Studies have shown that when you imagine moving, the same areas of your brain activate as if you are actually moving those specific muscles.[2] Through visualization, you are virtually exercising your body.

We are intending for you to have a tangible, physical response to the ideas in this book. The power of this story lies in the vividness of your imagination. Read slowly. Pause. Use all of your senses to experience the story. Imagine the changes in humidity. Feel the gentle breeze on your skin. Hear the soothing sound of the wind. Smell the fresh scent of the life around you. Use your vibrant imagination to experience every detail in this story.

Put yourself in the story. Try to experience every sensation in your body. If you feel like moving, do it! Trust your instincts. Imagine what it feels like to move through the story: your muscles warming and stretching... your breathing deepening... your heartbeat slowing as you deeply relax. Let these sensations come to you at the speed of thought. This isn't about concentrating as much as it is about experiencing.

Each time you practice visualizing this story, your experience will become more vibrant. Your body is your wilderness to explore and understand. Your mind is your canvas for new muscle memories.

The Reflections are our personal notes to you. They offer you insight into some of the concepts in the story. Use them to spark your own creative thoughts about connection and healing.

The Notes section is full of wonderful articles and books that we have selected for you. If you feel interested in a topic, we highly recommend you look at the notes to explore the topic further.

The Journal at the end of the book gives you an opportunity to enhance and deepen your meditation. We have asked you a few thought-provoking questions to help you get started. Feel free to write or draw. Journal as creatively as you are inspired. This is your time to dream of the supportive connections between your body and nature.

There is much to discover about your relationship with your body and the beautiful world around you. Find a comfortable place to relax and enjoy. Prepare to be transported to a setting where you can unwind, immersed in nature, and experience the unbridled freedom of the wild!

From Wellness To Oneness,

Erik and Faye
Your Virtual Massage Therapists

FROM WELLNESS TO ONENESS

Wherever you are,

however you feel,

whatever your state of wellness,

know that

healing is at hand.

Your body is always seeking balance

and looking for opportunities to restore.

Through wellness,

may you come to oneness

with your body,

your mind,

your spirit,

and the beautiful Earth that supports us all.

Introduction

When I was in college studying forestry, I had the privilege of working at the most remote ranger station in the United States. Rager Ranger Station was situated in the high desert of Eastern Oregon. The mystique of the antelope on the open plains, and the views that went on forever, were wildly inspiring to this native of New Orleans.

To this day, I go to the desert to clear my mind. I watch the clouds roll across the vast blue sky. I marvel at how the cold, clear nights can bring such warm days. In the high desert, I find myself in sync with nature's timing and my body's rhythms. Breathing the clean desert air refreshes my lungs. Sleeping soundly under the stars energizes me. Lifting my feet high to walk over the bumpy, rocky ground invigorates my whole body. I leave the high desert feeling stronger and more balanced.

I am excited to share these feelings with you. Enjoy communing with the high desert and feeling fully alive.

To experience the entire

NatureBody® Connection

scan this QR code

or go to

www.aquaterramassage.com / naturebodygift / highdesert

A gift for you, dear reader.

A special reading by the authors awaits you
at the link above.

CHAPTER ONE

Between Earth and Sky

STRETCHING AND GROUNDING

I am in the high desert, a wide-open country with expansive blue skies. I drink in the miles-long view over the ancient land. Wind blows across the plains dotted with juniper trees and sagebrush. My eyes stretch to see details on the distant horizon.

These high-elevation plains sit thousands of feet above sea level. Reaching out from the the base of glacial-peaked mountains, the high desert extends hundreds of miles. This land is arid and bright. The air is dry in the rain shadow of the mountains. The moisture from the sea is rung out of the air as it crosses the lofty mountain range.

These are the wild lands of the West, where antelope, deer and elk run free and bald eagles fly high.

I, too, feel wild and free in this vast, arid land.

Arching to Release Our Shoulders

*"I gaze into the vibrant blue sky,
the back of my neck lengthening into an arch."*

There is a wonderfully freeing feeling when we stretch up toward the sky. Arching upwards opens our chests and unwinds our rounded shoulders. This stretch helps encourage our bodies to a more natural, upright posture.

In our modern world, we spend many of our waking hours curled in front of computers, phones, books, and steering wheels. Our bodies adapt to these activities: our chest muscles tighten and our upper back muscles weaken. Our neck and shoulders are pulled forward off our center of gravity[3] in this hunched posture. Slouching can lead to back pain and stiffness in our neck and shoulders. It can restrict our breathing and make us more prone to headaches.

If your shoulders are curled forward, you can restore your balanced posture by standing tall and arching to the sky, as we visualized in this chapter. Engage your abs to support your spine in this arch. Lift your chest and spread your arms wide. Lengthen your neck and lightly pull your shoulder blades together. Breathe. Lowering your arms, you find yourself standing taller: your chest wider and your shoulders more open. You are reclaiming your natural, strong and confident[4] posture.

Good posture feels more comfortable, allows you to turn your head more freely and to breathe easier. As your upper body unwinds, it allows you to open your eyes to the world around you.

Century-old sagebrush shrubs add a pale green hue to the plains around me. Their weathered, sinewy forms contrast with their own new growth. Their fresh, tri-lobed leaves are soft and pliable. I pick a few leaves and roll them between my fingers. Their pungent fragrance tunes my senses to the land around me.

The fresh breeze is energized with the cleansing, grounding aroma of sage. The feeling of being in this clean mountain air is wonderful.

> *The air is so soft at this high elevation.*
> *I am uplifted by the feeling of freedom*
> *and aliveness here.*

> *I engage my core as I reach my hands up and out to the sky,*
> *and breathe.*

> *My chest opens.*

> *My body stretches long,*
> *all the way up from my toes.*

> *I gaze into the vibrant blue sky,*
> *the back of my neck lengthening into an arch.*

> *My throat softens.*

> *My shoulders and blades fall back and down.*

> *The energy my palms receive*
> *pours like a waterfall down to my center*
> *and through my feet.*

The Core of Movement

*"I imagine my body radiating out to infinity
while my balanced core is contained within a pinpoint."*

Our core lies at the heart of all we do. With a toned and balanced core, we can perform full body movements with confidence.

Our core muscles are the muscles between our diaphragm and our pelvic floor. The core enables us to arch, curl, and twist our spines. They distribute the effort between our upper and lower body. They stabilize our posture[6] and protect our low back when we do big, full-body movements, like twisting to reach the seatbelt, or picking something up off the floor. Be sure to engage your core before you arch, curl, twist or bend.

Imagine a seed with its precious life force encompassed in a protective outer shell. This seed is buried in your center of gravity, just below and behind your navel. Gather your muscles around this seed. Squeezing your center provides support and stability to your spine so that you have the freedom to move without injuring your low back.

By strongly holding this tiny space, large, full body movements become safe and grounded. A toned core is the foundation for your freedom of movement.

The sky is a rich blue on this beautiful day.

When I look straight up,
    the sky seems to deepen into a darker,
    richer shade of blue.

It feels as if I can almost see beyond the sky, into space.

A sense of connection pours through my being.

I imagine my body radiating out to infinity
    while my balanced core is contained
    within a pinpoint.

I feel as if I am blending into the sky.

The ancient earth grounds me.

The soles of my feet broadly connect with earth,
    allowing for my expansive stretch.

On Grounding

"I picture my exhales sinking deep into the land below my feet."

Grounding is a mindfulness technique that helps you connect to Earth's natural energy to replenish and calm yourself.[7] It brings you into the moment. Grounding helps you think more clearly and be more focused.

One way to practice grounding is to visualize energy from the sky pouring down through your head. Let the energy fill your body. Exhale the energy down your legs, through your feet, and all the way through the center of the earth. This establishes your connection from the sky.

Next, reverse this visualization. Inhale, pulling energy up from the Earth's core. Allow this earth energy to fill your body. Exhale this energy up and out to the sky. This establishes your connection from the earth.

Grounding is very important for caregivers and healers. By channeling Earth's unlimited energy, you can freely give to another without depleting your own energy.

Before you begin a new activity, grounding helps you let go of unnecessary thoughts, so you are more mindful of the task at hand. The feeling of presence that grounding offers can help you shake off performance anxiety.

Grounding is a way to gather your energy. Enjoy being the focus of energy from the sky above and the earth below. By grounding, you are fortifying your presence on the planet.

I imagine that I am magnetically connected
to the Earth's molten core.

I picture my exhales sinking deep
into the land below my feet.

I am stretching into the sky,
drinking the deep blue down into my body,
flushing it through the soil.

I am a conduit between Heaven and Earth.

Like a lightning rod,
I receive energy from the sky,
channel it through my body,
and send it plunging down into the earth.

My energy grounds into the earth
while rising up into the sky.

I feel focused and alive here in the high desert.

CHAPTER TWO

Spirit of the Antelope

AGILITY AND FREEDOM OF THE HIPS

Here on the high desert plateau, my brain relaxes as my eyes stretch to see as far as they can see. The land looks gentle and smooth at a distance. Assorted grasses and wildflowers wave together in the gentle breeze. I imagine herds of antelope racing freely across the plains.

I try to find my own graceful lope over the terrain, but what looks like smooth and gentle ground, is actually rocky. Lava rocks, many just small enough to be covered by sagebrush, pepper the grasslands. The crusty earth looks as though it is still healing from eons hence, when great lava flows oozed hundreds of miles across this land. They have left behind their geologic story.

The soil is not deep enough to cover the rock that dominates the landscape. The shallow soil and infrequent desert rain support only desert grasses, wildflowers, and the hardiest of trees and shrubs.

REFLECTION

The Grace of
an Antelope

"My walk over the plains becomes a high-stepped dance."

Antelope run smoothly and swiftly on rough and unpredictable terrain. They have a natural trot that can keep them moving lightly and easily across the landscape. Their legs open into a long stride as they increase their speed. With bursts of up to 55 miles per hour, soft pads on their hooves cushion their legs from the impact of running.

Visualize moving with the grace of an antelope.

Imagine your feet becoming more bouncy. Like the hooves of the antelope, you have pads in the balls and heels of your feet to cushion your steps and protect your joints.

Lift your knees high. Imagine you are stepping over rocks and shrubs. Let your hips open as you lengthen your stride, like the antelope trotting into a run. Keep your head high and aware as you move, scanning the horizon. Your upper body is relaxed and balanced on your hips. You are moving lightly and freely.

Enjoy your powerful springy legs and your relaxed upper body. Like an antelope, you can move gracefully over rough terrain.

I had imagined running free like the antelope: yet, even walking is challenging across this rugged terrain. To avoid tripping, I dig deeper into my imagination of the antelope.

My walk over the plains becomes a high-stepped dance.
Every step is deliberate.

I place my feet in the small
spaces between rocks.

I lift my knees high to
float over the sagebrush.

I step lightly on flat surfaces of the stones.
Sometimes my toes point forward.
Sometimes they angle to the side.

I skillfully pivot to the next step
as if I am prancing on small, delicate hooves.

I feel nimble.

I direct my movement from my strong center.
My hips swivel to keep my knees aligned.

My mind is pleasantly focused on my walk
across this uneven terrain.

I am mindful with each step,
present in this moment.

I begin to experience a rhythm in my walk.

Pivoting From Your Hips

*"I lift my knee, rotate my leg
and place my foot exactly in the spot I have chosen."*

Staying light on your feet can protect your joints.

If you turn your body too quickly without picking up your foot, it is easy to tweak your knee. Turning suddenly when your foot is planted can put unhealthy sheer force and torque on your knee joint.[8]

By picking up your foot before you turn your leg, you are freeing your joints. When you use the strength of your whole leg to help you pivot, you take strain off your knees and ankles.

Try this exercise to put more spring in your steps while protecting your joints. Pick up your foot, rotate your whole leg from the hip, then place your foot back down. Repeat this movement with the other leg, turning your body in a new direction. Feel your motions originating from your core. Your movements begin to feel like a dance.

Small changes in the way you move can make a big difference in the health and longevity of your joints.

By focusing on the ground several steps ahead,
   I am able to pick out my next step
   while keeping my head high.

I glance around,
   staying aware of my surroundings.

I lift my knee, rotate my leg
   and place my foot exactly in the spot I have chosen.

My hips are light and free in their movements.

The muscles of my legs wrap tautly around the bones
   to cushion my steps.

My feet prance nimbly over the sagebrush.

As my eyes get better at reading the terrain,
   I gradually pick up speed.

I accept the inevitability of unbalanced steps.
   It sometimes feels like my walk
   is more of a controlled fall.

My legs work quickly and succinctly.
   Keeping my balance becomes a workout
   for all of my muscles,
   especially the small muscles that surround my joints,
   essential to balance.

Finding Your Balance

*"As my body leans to the side, the tightening of my center,
a minor shift of my arm, a swivel of my hips,
a shrug of my shoulder brings me back upright."*

Developing your balance is a fun way to improve your overall fitness. When you challenge your balance, small muscles in your feet[9] and core coordinate their movements to keep you upright.[10] By doing balance exercises, you are stimulating and strengthening muscles that you might not even know you had.

To develop your ability to balance, try standing on one leg. Engage your core muscles. Distribute your weight between the ball and heel of your standing foot. Feel your foot adjusting to keep you upright. To further challenge your balance, close your eyes. This exercise develops your proprioception: your body's sense of where it is in space.[11]

Another way to improve your balance is to imagine you are walking on a tightrope. Engage your core muscles. Walk with your arms outstretched, placing one foot directly in front of the other, heel to toe. Look forward, fixing your eyes on a specific point. Try the same exercise with your arms down by your sides.

With all balance exercises, your core is key. Simply focus on keeping your core engaged. This one thought simplifies your effort. No matter what balancing act you are trying to achieve, the result is the same: you are floating your core over the earth.

As my body leans to the side,
the tightening of my center,
a minor shift of my arm,
a swivel of my hips,
a shrug of my shoulder,
brings me back upright.

My body is becoming better at counterbalancing
to keep me upright.
It strives to float my core smoothly across the earth.

I find that my legs, hips, even my back and arms
are being worked in an unusually satisfying way.

My limbs instinctively adjust as I stabilize my center.

In the high desert, walking is a full body exercise. I feel like a tightrope walker striving to keep their feet under them. The dynamic and varied muscles of my legs and hips serve to float my core over my feet.

I am not running freely across the open grasslands as I had imagined. And yet I feel complete freedom here.

My legs are fully expressing themselves,
using each and every muscle,
as they carry me across this landscape.

I am grateful to feel the free dance of movement
in this wild, untamed land.

The spirit of the antelope is being expressed through me.

CHAPTER THREE

Wisdom of the Land

AGING WITH GRACE

This is ancient country. Perennial vegetation lives long in this arid landscape. Century-old sagebrush thrives here. Ancient-looking lichens paint the rocks in patterns that remind me of prehistoric rock art, as if the lichens are trying to tell me the story of this land.

I find myself searching the terrain for clues, trying to read the story of the land. I look intently to soak in its knowledge.

The land has aged and cracked with time. Where the thick basalt rock fractured, water concentrated, and canyons formed. The soil grew deep. Life became plentiful. The canyons have become wildlife highways, abundant with huckleberry bushes and other lush edible forage. Cottonwoods and quaking aspen trees grow in the center of these hidden oases where intermittent water flows. Towering ponderosa pine forests thrive in the shelter of

The Strength of a Tree

"My abdominal muscles hold my body tight to my spine to make me taller."

As a tree is shielded with bark, we are covered with protective muscle. Muscles both large and small surround and support every part of our body. We are wrapped in muscle.

A tree's bark, *phloem*, protects the living layer, *cambium*, just inside its bark.[12] Like a tree, our muscles protect our most important living layer: our spinal cord.

Our spinal cord is the electrical highway of communication between our brain and the rest of our body. This delicate cord is covered by layers of protective sheathing, and is lubricated and cushioned by cerebrospinal fluid.[13] Our vertebral bones surround and protect our spinal cord, while their soft, intervertebral discs cushion its structure. The layers of security around our most precious conductor of thought keep us healthy and strong.

By strengthening the muscles of our core and torso, we build another layer of support around our spine, as if we were strong trees. Allow yourself to stand as tall as a magnificent tree. Your core muscles work together to keep your spine erect.[14] Feel your muscles wrapping around your strong center as you rise up toward the sun. You are enfolding your spine in layers of protection, taking pressure off your back and supporting this essential neurological structure.

these canyons.

The grandest of the ponderosa pine trees tower proudly, living nearly 1000 years. These dignified grandfathers of the high desert show their age with grace. Their straight, magnificent golden trunks are the sign that they have reached maturity. As they age, they begin to smell like vanilla.

> I press my nose up to the bark
>   of a yellow-bellied ancient ponderosa,
>   and inhale the delightfully sweet scent.

These trees become continually more beautiful through the years, their statuesque presence filling out over time. Their needles are continuously discarded and renewed and look as fresh as they did in the tree's infancy.

> I would like to age as gracefully
>   as the stately ponderosa pine.

> I imagine my own body
>   rising tall out of my core.

> My abdominal muscles
>   hold my body tight to my spine
>   to make me taller.

> I engage my core, lengthening my torso
>   and reaching out of the top of my head.
>   I feel the pressure being taken off my spine.

> I feel the discs between my vertebrae
>   opening and rehydrating.

On Aging

"I appreciate the weathering and aging of my form."

We become more unique as we age. Rather than seeing aging as a deterioration of your body, consider that your life's experience is sculpting and refining your body.

Our hobbies and careers shape our bodies. Our muscles strengthen or weaken to accommodate our activities. Through the years, habitual patterns in the way we walk, sit, gesture and move influence our structure. Our tissues conform to support us.

Challenging yourself with new activities not only builds new connections in your brain, it also strengthens your muscles with new patterns of movement. Your body adapts by creating new muscle memories: reawakening muscles that have weakened over time, and stretching muscles that have become tight through the years.

Massaging your muscles can help maintain their pliability and ability to adapt. Staying hydrated has also been linked to healthier aging.[15]

No matter what age you are, your body is always trying to respond and adapt to the challenges you put in front of it. By trying new hobbies, learning new skills, and caring for yourself, you are helping your body thrive as you age.

My head reaches toward the sky
*   while my breath floats me yet higher.*

My posture feels more stable and balanced.

I imagine myself walking stately and tall
*   like a dignified ponderosa.*

I walk toward the junipers in the open sage flats. Juniper trees can live 700 years. They seem like they have stories to tell with their twisted, contorted forms. They are crooked and gnarled, and yet the junipers have found balance in their seeming imperfection. Each tree's unique form tells the story of its life and the challenging conditions it has survived.

Even in the harshest seasons, the junipers persist and bestow their gifts.

Junipers live in exposed scabland. They root in the shallow-soiled sage flats, away from the protection of the forest. They offer shelter in the midst of strong, icy windstorms. They provide shade while the sun bakes their branches. They produce succulent berries for wildlife in the midst of long droughts.

My body has also weathered the storms of my life
*   and found ways to adapt and be whole.*

I appreciate the weathering and aging of my form.

I have unique gifts and strengths to share with others:
*   gifts that could only be obtained*
*   by living through my life's challenges.*

Nurturing Yourself

"I nurture myself so that I may give back to the world."

Treating others as you would treat yourself, begins by treating *yourself* as you would treat others. Nurturing yourself can (and should!) be simple and joyful. By starting with your own self care, you create the energy that you wish to share.

Drinking water is one of the most powerful things you can do for your body. It helps you think more clearly, boosts your energy, and supports healthy digestion.[16]

Eating nourishing foods gives you energy and keeps your skin supple and radiant. Oiling your skin protects the largest organ of your body, and is a wonderful way to add self massage to your daily routine.

Stretching and moving warms your muscles and stimulates circulation. Go for a walk. Spend time in nature.

Make time for a good night's sleep. Sleeping boosts our memory and learning, and helps us live long, healthy lives.[17] Practice gratitude. Give thanks each day and night. An attitude of gratitude puts you into a healing state of mind.[18]

When you nurture yourself, you have more energy to do the things you find important in the world. You can do more for the people you love. Your mission and purpose begin by caring for yourself.

My youthful strength
  has been replaced with a tempered determination,
  and an appreciation of my wonderful body.

I relish my imperfections and feel grateful
  to move, to stretch, to be alive.

My muscles spiral around bone
  to keep me upright and moving on the earth.

I stretch and strengthen them
  to fine-tune my balance,
  and help me win the battle against gravity.

I drink water so my body can renew itself and stay supple.
  Water is life.

I eat to nourish my body.
  I oil my skin to protect it from the elements.
  I nurture myself so that I may give back to the world.

I am grateful that my own body
  has formed in the perfect way
  to function and protect me
  as I travel along life's meandering path.

My imperfections and scars tell my own life story.

I strive to be as tall and magnificent as a ponderosa pine.
  I honor my body, knowing it is continually
  adapting to life's challenges,
  like the resilient juniper.

CHAPTER FOUR

Wind Song and Cloud Stories

BREATHING MEDITATION

Wind blows across the open land. Sweetened with sage and juniper berry, it drifts across the highlands and into the tops of the ponderosa pines. Their crowns dance and their needles sing softly with the breeze.

I watch and listen to the waves of wind swirling over the landscape and inspiring my joyful spirit. It is as if the voices of the desert are carried on the wind.

The breeze subsides and stillness returns. Birds begin to sing.

I close my eyes to listen.

I am surrounded by the music of birdsong.
  It delights my senses.

On Breathing Freely

"I breathe in deeply to feel connected to the clouds."

There are as many ways to breathe as there are shapes of clouds in the sky. From yoga to pilates, from weightlifting to meditation, from singing to psychology, most forms of expression teach methods of breathing that enhance our experience.

Breathing can also affect our energy and mood. Two prominent techniques to balance our energy and influence our mood are "ocean breathing" and "box breathing."

Ocean breathing builds our inner heat and boosts our vitality.[19] Take a long, calming breath in through your nose. Open your mouth and exhale, making the "haaa" sound of the ocean. Taking a few ocean breaths warms your body, uplifts your spirit, and focuses your energy.

"Box breathing" calms your nervous system.[20] Begin by exhaling to the count of four, and then hold your breath out for the count of four. Inhale to the count of four and hold your breath in to the count of four. Box breathing slows the pace of your breath, pulling you out of the fight-or-flight response, and back into the rest-and-digest mode.

Skilled breathing can help you feel and perform better: physically, mentally and energetically.

I feel their lively chorus soothe and heal me.

Their intermittent calls
    bring patience to my anticipation.

I gaze up at the clouds dancing across the bright blue sky. The clouds are shaped by the wind over the landscape. With long, sweeping brushstrokes, the clouds speak of the wide-open fetch of the grasslands.

I breathe in deeply to feel connected to the clouds.

My lungs are open and free.

Mountains have studded this open plain. Warm winds rise up the mountainside from low elevations to cool altitudes above. Huge, billowing clouds form over the mountains.

Across the blue sky,
    puffy cumulus clouds
    illustrate the stories of daydreams.

I imagine I see these daydreams
    parading across the sky
    as they twist and form different shapes and patterns.

I see the movement of the wind in the texture of the clouds. High above the puffy cumulus clouds, cirrus clouds form an icy veil across the top of our atmosphere. Dominant winds paint feathery brushstrokes through the cirrus clouds in one direction. Secondary wind patterns skid across these smooth lines, creating crosshatched patterns.

Far in the distant horizon, lens-shaped lenticular clouds dome over lofty peaks of mountaintops.

The Breathing Planet

"The sky is offering me breath."

Half the oxygen on Earth is formed in the ocean, most of it by tiny photosynthetic algae called phytoplankton.[21] The other half of Earth's oxygen is created by our forests.

The circulation of oxygen over our planet ebbs and flows with the seasons. Each spring and summer, as new leaflets unfurl, the forests turn green and photosynthesize. Oxygen flourishes with this seasonal flush of new growth in the forests and the seasonal bloom of phytoplankton in the oceans. When photosynthesis subsides in winter, oxygen levels decrease.

While the northern hemisphere welcomes the flush of new spring growth and the renewal of oxygen, autumn leaves fall in the southern hemisphere and oxygen levels subside. Like a lava lamp, oxygen swells and shrinks throughout the seasons across our planet. Our living planet breathes.

NASA created a beautiful time-lapse video showing the seasonal fluctuation of oxygen in our forests and oceans.[22,23] We see oxygen flow from the northern hemisphere to the southern, rhythmically, flushing through the great forests and throughout the seas.

The breath of oxygen ebbs and flows around the earth, bathing us all in life-giving atmosphere.

The clouds are showing me the story of the wind and the lay of the land. I watch and imagine the invisible dance of wind at each elevation, down to my level.

The grasses dance below me and I am buoyed by the movement I see.

> I imagine myself light of foot,
>   dancing in the grasses
>   with my head in the clouds.

> I turn into the wind and feel it blow into my nostrils,
>   my throat.

> The sky is offering me breath.

> I allow it to fill my lungs,
>   receiving the healing spirit of the high desert.

> I close my eyes to feel the wind more vividly.

> My body feels light and airy.

> I imagine dissolving into the wind
>   and becoming one with the open skies.

CHAPTER FIVE

Transition To Evening

FULL BODY MEDITATION

This beautiful day in the high desert started magically, with an elk bugling on the morning mist. The frosty chill of the morning transformed into a warm bright day.

> *I witnessed the desert come into full detail*
> *from the dark shadows of morning*
> *to the rosy welcoming of the day.*

The grace of the sun shone brilliantly upon everything. The midday sun blazed across the land. The clean air allowed me to see details all the way to the horizon. I could see for miles.

Afternoon shadows brought color and crisp detail to the sparse grasses and lichen-textured rocks. Desert sage and bitter brush, kinnikinnick, and wild onions all displayed their brilliant detail in the angled sun. The sun slowly moved across the sky. The shadows continued to lengthen.

The Ideal Bedroll

"A thick, inviting blanket of soft pine needles covers the ground underneath its canopy."

If you ever get a chance to lie down under a pine tree, you will find the thick bed of pine needles provides a lovely, soft cushion for your body. Some of the original mattresses were stuffed with pine straw.[24]

Many of us are in search of a mattress that will help us sleep deeply so we can wake up feeling mentally rested and physically energized. A great mattress cushions and supports us, allowing our muscles to let go completely as we sleep.

A soft and pillowy top layer is important in a good mattress because it reduces the pressure on our hips, sacrum, and shoulders. Extra cushion allows our blood to continue flowing through our capillaries[25] so we do not need to turn over as often. The soft top fills the spaces in our natural curves, gently holding our body as we sleep.

A supportive under layer is important as well. A firm mattress supports our skeleton, so that we do not bend out of alignment as the mattress sags. When our skeletal frame is aligned and supported, our muscles are free to relax.

A comfortable mattress supports our structure and cushions our curves, allowing our sleep to be deeply restful and healing.

Now, as afternoon softens into sunset, crickets begin their evening chorus. The breeze continues to swell in the air around me.

In the evening as the sun is setting, the angled rays glow in the grasses. The soft, golden light makes everything look gentle and even. The rocks seem to disappear in the tranquil evening light. The sky is a dusky pink, full of milky clouds poured across the horizon. I look across a field of grasses, each blade, pink and golden, reflecting the color of sunset.

The soft breeze gently touches my skin.

I am bathed in the calm that permeates the landscape.

I slowly walk to a ponderosa pine. A thick, inviting blanket of soft pine needles covers the ground underneath its canopy.

I lie down in the soft pine needles. Above me, small birds rustle toward their roosts as they settle in for the evening. Golden-pink clouds curve gently in the sky.

This large ponderosa smells of vanilla.

I deeply inhale its scent, filling my senses.

As my body relaxes and widens across the bed of pine needles, I allow my breath to expand my back.

My ribcage widens away from my spine.

I enjoy the gentle ebb and flow of my breathing.

Effortless Breathing

"My abdomen rises and falls gently.
I breathe as softly as a cloud floating across the sky."

A relaxed breath can feel effortless and easy. When you watch a young child sleep, you see their breathing slow, becoming nearly imperceptible as their body relaxes. Their breathing is easy and natural.

Where many of us feel that we need to take full, deep breaths to relax, relaxing can be as easy as softening your breath.

Visualize your precious inner child. Allow your breath to become softer and quieter, like a sleeping infant.

Feel your breath enter your nose, filling your sinuses. Notice your abdomen expand with your inhale and soften with your exhale. Take your time with your breath. Feel your body relax.

As your breathing becomes more effortless, imagine a wave of relaxation pouring down your body. Visualize it flowing down your head, your neck, your shoulders, arms, your hands and out your fingertips. Feel its innocent splendor pour down your spine, your hips, your feet and your toes.

Invite relaxation throughout your body. Let your easy, effortless breathing fill you with relaxation.

I draw my breath deeper down to my pelvis.
My hips widen and lengthen
with the support of the ground.

My back sinks into the pine straw,
and my abdomen feels longer and more supple.

The backs of my knees open to the earth.

My heels sink as my arches relax.

I spread my toes
and feel the gentle breeze between them.

My abdomen rises and falls gently.
I breathe as softly as a cloud floating across the sky.

My chest opens wide
as my shoulders and arms relax.

The soft bed below me gives me a feeling of floating.

My throat softens
as my jaw releases
and my tongue relaxes.

My scalp eases and my ears draw back toward the earth.

My face is free of expression, open to the sky.

On Eternity

"I am one with this ancient land, experiencing eternity."

I am nourished by the natural world. The earth gives me the simple and vital elements that nurture me: food, water, fresh air, shelter, solace, excitement, and creative expression. From the gaseous atmosphere above, through the living biosphere, into the solidity of the earth's crust, and down deep to the liquid, molten core, my body is intimately connected to the planet. The living earth replenishes me, body and soul.

Sprites of lightning replenish the protective ozone around our planet. Lightning purifies the atmosphere for a clean breath of air. Bathing in cool water relaxes my nervous system. Warm sunlight comforts my muscles. Vital, nourishing foods grow around me in the rich soil. Fresh breezes cleanse my energy and uplift my thoughts. Vast landscapes lure me into mediative mindfulness.

These thoughts bring me into a deep appreciation of my home here on Earth. When I spend time in nature, my thoughts take on a positive note, leading me to places greater than myself. I come to understand that I am part of a great and timeless power.

In fleeting moments, I recognize that am living in a veritable Heaven on Earth. I understand, in these moments, that I am experiencing eternity. I am thankful for these moments of clarity. I live with gratitude for these moments and seek to create them again, for myself and others.

I feel my silent breath,
   rising,
   falling,
   in,
   out...

The chirping of the birds and the chittering of the squirrels fade into the twilight. The evening song of crickets, the occasional hooting of an owl, and the yipping chorus of distant coyotes herald the peace of nighttime. The desert night is born anew.

I am one with this ancient land,
   experiencing eternity.

CHAPTER SIX

Gratitude

A BLESSING FROM THE HIGH DESERT

T hank you for joining me on this journey through ancient land. Since the dawn of time, geology has written its ancient story across the changing landscape. Until we meet again,

May the strength of the sun encourage you to shine brightly.

May the spirit of the antelope inspire your run.

May you hear wisdom in the wind.

May you find peace
through your connection with nature.

May the moisture of clouds
  nourish your growth and imagination.

May the ponderosa pine remind you to stand tall,
  firm in your magnificence.

Dream on, Tranquil Wanderer.

Acknowledgments

Thank you to our dear friend, Herschel, for the wonderful campouts under the stars and early mornings in the sagebrush.

My great-grandfather, Dr. Clyde Bollinger, spent his lifetime studying weather patterns and making connections with the universe. His work correlating the influence of solar flares to Earth's climate patterns has inspired me to continue to look for connections in nature.

The wonderful people I met at Rager Ranger Station helped broaden my horizons and expand my outlook on life. My seasons in the high plains of Central Oregon inspire me to dream bigger.

Thank you to Marty Ryan and his *Love Your Guts* seminars on abdominal palpation. He introduced us to the beauty of our abdomen and its visceral magnificence, and to Gil Hedley.

Gil Hedley's lessons on anatomy blend a special reverence for the human form with teachings of its structures. We have deeply appreciated his thoughtful lectures and respectful purpose.

In the Thomas Condon visitor center at the John Day Fossil Beds National Monument, there is a fossil museum that offers a fantastic geologic perspective of the high desert. The museum brings you back to the times when the desert was a semitropical paradise, where giant rhinoceros-like creatures and tiny horses roamed among among banana plants and under magnolia trees, and the song of cicadas filled the humid forest.

Notes

1. "What is Imagery?" *Johns Hopkins Medicine*, 2003, www.hopkinsmedicine.org/health/wellness-and-prevention/imagery.

2. Lohr, Jim. "Can Visualizing Your Body Doing Something Help You Learn to Do It Better?" *Scientific American*, 1 May 2015, www.scientificamerican.com/article/can-visualizing-your-body-doing-something-help-you-learn-to-do-it-better.

3. "Upper-Crossed Syndrome." *Physiopedia*, www.physiopedia.com/Upper-Crossed_Syndrome. Accessed 8 February 2023.

4. Schmidt, Kendall Lou. "Posture Power: How To Correct Your Body's Alignment." *Bodybuilding*, 14 June 2017, www.bodybuilding.com/content/posture-power-how-to-correct-your-body-alignment.html.

5. "The Real-World Effects of Strengthening Your Core." *Harvard Health Publishing,* 24 January 2012, www.health.harvard.edu/healthbeat/the-real-world-benefits-of-strengthening-your-core.

6. "Core Muscles." *Physiopedia,* www.physio-pedia.com/Core_Muscles. Accessed 10 February 2023.

7. Gold, Jamie. "The Wellness Design Benefits Of Grounding." *Forbes,* 21 September 2021, www.forbes.com/sites/jamiegold/2021/09/21/the-wellness-design-benefits-of-grounding.

8. "Torn Meniscus." *Mayo Clinic,* 2023. www.mayoclinic.org/diseases-conditions/torn-meniscus/symptoms-causes/syc-20354818. Accessed 27 January 2023.

9. Gudmestad, Julie. "Focus on Your Feet: How to Improve Balance and Prevent Injuries." *Yoga Journal,* 28 August 2007, www.yogajournal.com/teach/anatomy-yoga-practice/feet-first.

10. Freytag, Chris. "5 Balance Exercises to Boost Stability and Performance." *Very Well Fit,* 5 October 2022, www.verywellfit.com/exercises-for-better-balance-3498203.

11. Inverarity, Laura. "An Overview of Proprioception." *Very Well Health,* 22 May 2022, www.verywellhealth.com/proprioception-2696141.

12. "Anatomy of a Tree." *Arbor Day Foundation,* www.arborday.org/trees/treeguide/anatomy.cfm. Accessed 30 January 2023.

13. Sendic, Gordana. "Cerebrospinal Fluid Flow." *Kenhub,* 22 July 2022, www.kenhub.com/en/library/anatomy/circulation-of-the-cerebrospinal-fluid.

14. "Why a Strong Core Can Help Reduce Low Back Pain." *Cleveland Clinic,* 29 May 2020, health.clevelandclinic.org/strong-core-best-guard-back-pain.

15. "Good Hydration Linked to Healthy Aging." *National Heart, Lung and Blood Institute,* 2 January 2023, www.nhlbi.nih.gov/news/2023/good-hydration-linked-healthy-aging.

16. Leech, Joe. "7 Science-Based Health Benefits of Drinking Enough Water." *Healthline,* 30 June 2020, www.healthline.com/nutrition/7-health-benefits-of-water#The-bottom-line.

17. "Benefits of Sleep." *Division of Sleep Medicine at Harvard Medical School,* healthysleep.med.harvard.edu/healthy/matters/benefits-of-sleep. Accessed 27 January 2023.

18. Firestone, Lisa. "The Healing Power of Gratitude." *Psychology Today,* 19 November 2015, www.psychologytoday.com/us/blog/compassion-matters/201511/the-healing-power-gratitude.

19. Pizer, Ann. "How to Do Ocean Breath (Ujjayi Pranayama) in Yoga." *Very Well Fit,* 30 June 2020, verywellfit.com/ocean-breath-ujjayi-pranayama-3566763.

20. Stinson, Adrienne. "What is Box Breathing?" *Medical News Today,* 6 January 2023, www.medicalnewstoday.com/articles/321805.

21. "How Much Oxygen Comes from the Ocean?" *National Ocean Service,* oceanservice.noaa.gov/facts/ocean-oxygen.html. Accessed 27 January 2023.

22. Pidcock, Roz. "Video: NASA Satellites Show Our 'Breathing' Planet in Action." *CarbonBrief,* 17 November 2015, www.carbonbrief.org/video-nasa-satellites-show-our-breathing-planet-in-action.

23. "Watching Earth Breathe: the Seasonal Vegetation Cycle and Carbon Dioxide." *NASA Jet Propulsion Laboratory,* 28 November 2012, www.jpl.nasa.gov/videos/watching-earth-breathe-the-seasonal-vegetation-cycle-and-carbon-dioxide.

24. "Pine Straw Mattress Factory." *Anchor, A North Carolina History Online Resource,* www.ncpedia.org/media/pine-straw-mattress-factory. Accessed 31 January 2023.

25. Watson, Stephanie. "The Best Mattress for a Better Night's Sleep." *WebMD,* 3 March 2014, www.webmd.com/sleep-disorders/features/best-mattress-good-nights-sleep.

MEDITATION

Journal

This journal gives you a place to reflect on your experience as you read and meditate. With every meditation, your library of personal affirmations can grow. Some thoughts you might want to record, in words or drawings, are:

What physical sensations did you notice in your body before, during and after the meditation? What changes would you like to make in your posture?

How would you like to move more freely? Visualize moving without restriction. Is there an animal you admire for its freedom of movement?

When you think of the ponderosa pine and juniper trees, how do you relate to your own maturing body?

Now that you are more aware of your breathing, what connections do you feel with the earth and the sky?

May the

STRENGTH

of the

SUN

encourage you

to shine brightly.

"I FEEL WILD AND FREE IN THESE VAST, ARID GRASSLANDS."

MEDITATION

Out in nature, we experience the wildness of our bodies. We move and breathe with the wind, the grass, the rolling hills.

You are not disconnected from nature. You *are* nature, and your body is your conduit to the wild world.

~

May the
SPIRIT
of the
ANTELOPE
inspire your run.

"GRASSES OF MANY VARIETIES WAVE TOGETHER IN THE GENTLE BREEZE."

MEDITATION

Nature shows us the power of non-resistance in many ways. Seeing soft grasses in the breeze reminds us to move and flow, to be strong, yet flexible, bending with the wind.

~

May you

HEAR
WISDOM

in the wind.

"MY ENERGY GROUNDS INTO THE
EARTH WHILE IT RISES UP INTO
THE SKY. I FEEL FOCUSED AND
ALIVE."

MEDITATION

With your feet on the ground and your head in the clouds, you are connected to all that is. Dream big as you deepen your roots.

~

May you
FIND
PEACE
through

your connection

with nature.

"THE SOFT BREEZE GENTLY
TOUCHES MY SKIN. I AM BATHED
IN THE CALM THAT PERMEATES
THE LANDSCAPE."

MEDITATION

When you close your eyes, you can feel the breeze more vividly. Be in the moment. Allow yourself to be consciously connected to the living world around you.

~

May the

MOISTURE

of the

CLOUDS

nourish your growth

and imagination.

"I SEE THE MOVEMENT OF THE
WIND IN THE TEXTURE OF THE
CLOUDS."

MEDITATION

A cloudscape tells a story. Watch the textures above. Notice the layers of clouds in the sky. Your exhales billow out to join the story of the clouds.

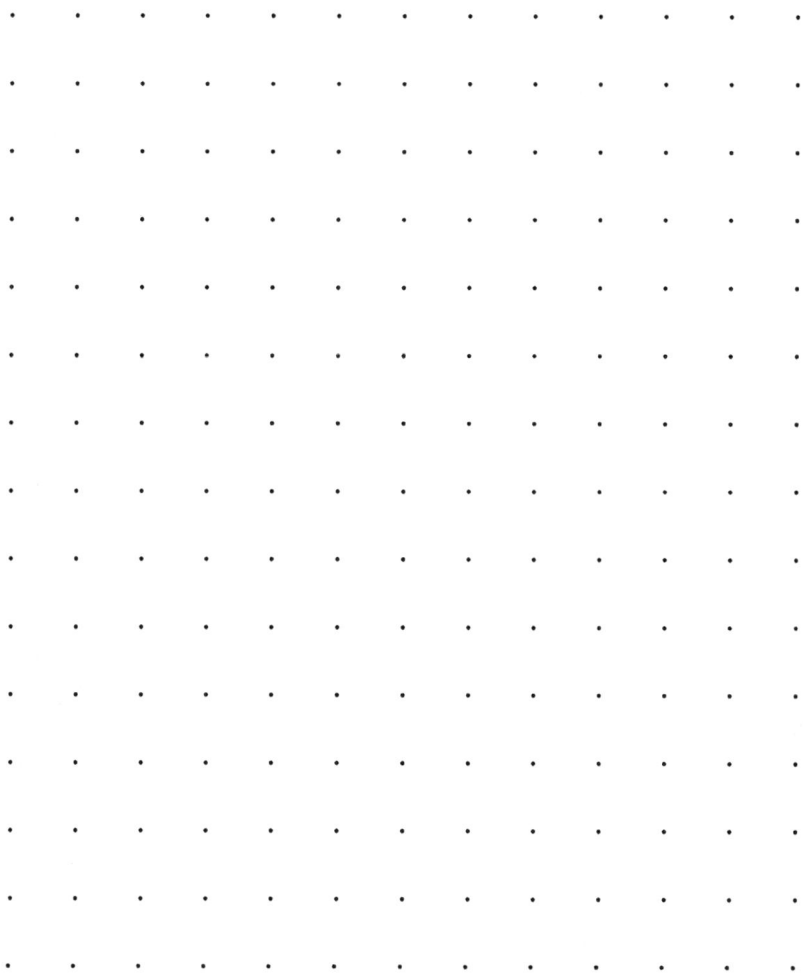

~

"EVEN UP ON THE PLATEAUS THE
ABUNDANCE OF LIFE IS EASY TO
SEE."

MEDITATION

All around the world, even in the most challenging environments, life finds a way to exist. How has your body adapted to your life's challenges? How has your body helped you to thrive?

~

May the

PONDEROSA PINE

remind you

to stand tall,

firm in your

MAGNIFICENCE.

"THE FRESH BREEZE IS ENERGIZED
WITH THE GROUNDING,
CLEANSING AROMA OF SAGE."

MEDITATION

When you walk in nature, you are surrounded by medicinal plants and herbs. Next time you go out in nature, notice the variety of plants and shrubs around you. Inhale the wild scents of the air. Embrace the magic of Earth's healing nature.

You are part of this magic. You are part of Earth's healing nature.

~

"I TRUST THAT MY OWN BODY HAS FORMED IN THE PERFECT WAY TO FUNCTION AND PROTECT ME AS I TRAVEL ALONG LIFE'S PATH."

MEDITATION

Our bodies are always adapting: responding to our activities and our experiences. They tune our balance to meet our needs.

When you exercise, your body responds by strengthening your muscles. When you sit for extended periods, your body shortens some muscles and lengthens others. If you become injured, your body tightens the muscles around the injury to protect you.

Sometimes our bodies get sore. Sometimes they don't perform as quickly or strongly as we would like. But our bodies are dedicated to us and all that we want to achieve. Having a positive attitude can tune our mind to work in harmony with our bodies.

~

BLESSING
FROM THE HIGH DESERT

May the

STRENGTH OF THE SUN
encourage you to shine brightly.

May the

SPIRIT OF THE ANTELOPE
inspire your run.

May you hear

WISDOM IN THE WIND.

May you

FIND PEACE
through your connection with nature.

May the

MOISTURE OF THE CLOUDS
nourish your growth and imagination.

May the

PONDEROSA PINE
remind you to stand tall,
firm in your

MAGNIFICENCE.

About the Authors

Born and raised in New Orleans, Erik Krippner grew up with a po'boy in his hand and a song in his heart. As a boy, he spent his summers swimming, hiking, fishing, and sailing. After becoming an Eagle Scout, Erik dreamed of answering the call to "Go West, young man." He earned a Bachelor of Science degree in Forestry from Louisiana State University. Following his passion for adventure, Erik found his way to the mountains of the Pacific Northwest, his home to this day. After working in the forests of Oregon, Washington, Idaho, Alaska, Georgia, and Louisiana, Erik decided to focus his love of natural sciences on the study of human body through massage therapy.

Faye grew up in Oregon surrounded by family and old growth coastal forests. She spent many childhood weekends cross-country skiing, hunting for mushrooms, exploring coastal tide pools, and searching for crawdads in the Siuslaw River. Her love of books deepened when she became the editor of her high school and college's literary journals. Upon earning her Bachelor of Arts degree in Mathematics with honors from the Robert D. Clark Honors College at the University of Oregon, Faye became a technical writer and web developer. The whisper of a deeper purpose ignited her to study massage, where she met Erik.

Erik and Faye became friends in massage school at the East West College of the Healing Arts, in Portland, Oregon. In 2003, they founded Aqua Terra Massage, a therapeutic massage studio for friends and couples. Since then, they have practiced therapeutic massage together, side by side. They have spent years immersed in the study of massage, serving thousands of clients.

Faye and Erik have spent years exploring and writing about our beautiful world. They have sailed the blue waters of Fiji's Koro Sea, kayaked New Zealand's Marlborough Sound, and stargazed among the giraffes and elephants in Botswana. They have hiked the Appalachian Trail and paddled the tidally-influenced Columbia River in the Pacific Northwest. They have seen orca whales swim right under their kayaks, locked eyes with wild lions, and played hide-and-seek with an octopus. They have hiked thousands of miles together, kayaked and sailed hundreds, and spent countless evenings camping under the stars.

With a commitment to bringing more love and kindness
to this beautiful world, we offer this book to you.

www.aquaterramassage.com

www.ingramcontent.com/pod-product-compliance
Lightning Source LLC
Chambersburg PA
CBHW071404050426
42335CB00063B/1630